FAT

2

FIT

HOW I LOST 54 LBS. IN 42 DAYS

Chandler G. Coleman

ISBN: 0692219625
ISBN-13: 978-0692219621

DEDICATION

I would like to dedicate this book in memory of my parents, the late Garland and Mary Coleman, who taught me how to take control of my destiny and taught me the difference between handling life and not allowing life to handle me.

This book is also dedicated to my wonderful wife, Charita, and my son Chandler II, whom I hold dear to my heart. Both are great sources of inspiration and encouragement.

Last but not least, I dedicate this book to all of those who God used to persuade me to write this book. Timing is everything.

FAT 2 FIT

Table of Contents

BONUS:
- SAMPLE MENU
- WORKOUT REGIMEN
- WORDS OF MOTIVATION
- TESTIMONIALS
- QUICK TIPS
- *more....*

BEFORE AND AFTER MY CHANGE

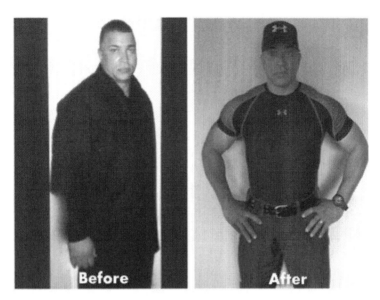

IN 42 DAYS I LOST 54 LBS.

INTRODUCTION

In 2002, my journey began. I decided to take control of my health. I found myself in the gym daily talking to trainers, trying to learn more about exercise. However, I soon realized they all had various advice and techniques which only frustrated and overwhelmed me. So I had to study training for myself. And because I thought I knew what it meant to eat right, I ate based on my limited knowledge. That is why reading this whole book is critical for you to succeed in your health and weight goal endeavors.

My favorite book in the Bible is 2 Timothy. In this book I found my guidance in chapter 2 verse 15 which states: "Study to show thyself approved unto God, a workman that need not to be ashamed, rightly dividing the word of truth." This word from God was confirmation that in order to succeed in this area of my life I had to study nutrition and fitness.

My desire is that the content of this book will change your life, increase the quality of your living, and teach you to value the most valuable asset you will ever own in this life, your body.

FORWARD

I met with a doctor from John Hopkins who did nutrition part time away from his duties at the hospital so that I could simply share my P.E.R. Fat Loss System. I thought he could expand my horizon in knowledge to maximize the potential of my system to help others. After I shared my system with him, he looked at me and said, "It seems like you have found the secret." My question is why does it have to be a secret? It could be if people really knew the power of food and its ability to heal the body most doctors and pharmaceutical companies would go out of business. I could understand why certain doctors would want this to remain a secret! Instead of medicines, food can be used as an alternative to restore the body. Yes medicines treat symptoms, but most have side effects, whereas food heals the body with minimal or no side effects. We have to be serious and take control of our destiny when it pertains to our health.

PREVIEW

I remember a gentlemen told me, "If a person cannot accomplish their weight goal desires on your plan they may as well quit." I believe he said this after seeing the menu and all the food choices it included. He was truly blown away! I tell folks I eat what I want and that is not a play on words. I simply eat what I want, but because I do not have the food cravings I use to have, I can eat what I want; just not all the time. When I eat something off the P.E.R. menu I know what foods to combine with whatever I am eating to counter the effect of medium or high glycemic foods to keep my body from going into fat storing mode. Balancing your food options by pairing what you want with what you need is important.

CHAPTER 1

THE JOURNEY BEGINS

Some of the information in this book is repetitious, but I think repetition is good for you to better retain the information, so keep that in mind as you continue to read this book.

During a journey there is a point that you start from, the course, and then your destination. Have you ever been going somewhere, got lost, and turned to someone for directions, and as soon as they started giving you directions you knew at that point if that person knew what they were talking about or not? That's what happened to some people when they started on this journey of health; they simply asked the wrong person for directions. Then there are those who not only know how to get you to a particular destination, but they have taken that same journey. These individuals are so convincing you can hear it in them when they are giving you the instructions or directions towards a certain destination. Why? Because, again, they have been there, and because they know where you want to go and are interested in you getting there. They will say, "Look follow me." This is one way to be reassured that you will reach your destination. Today I am that person giving you the direction where you want to go. I have been there and I know exactly how to get you there, just follow my lead.

I began my day at 5:30 am, getting to the gym at 6 am to work out. My workouts consisted of one hour circuit training, but first I would do ten minutes on the treadmill to warm the muscles up. Circuit training is when you work multiple muscles together with very limited breaks in between sets. I would work out the biceps, back (or triceps) chest, shoulders, and train my legs on a day by themselves. During circuit training I had 60 second breaks in between sets that would cause my heart rate to remain elevated while training my body to burn the most fat and build muscle. I was training and eating healthier, so I thought. I was excited because my diligence seemed to be paying off. Then it happened, the unimaginable, the unthinkable, I injured myself. I was hurt and could not exercise. Soon the 50 pounds I had lost came back, plus some. What happened? I thought I knew all I needed to know to accomplish my weight loss goals. I became quite discouraged; thinking of all the hard work I had put into getting fit just to realize it was temporary. My thought was I could not afford to put that kind of time and energy into something that was not permanent. I know some of you can relate and that is why it is imperative you continue to read this book if you want to succeed in your health. 3John 1:2 "Beloved, I wish above all things that thou mayest prosper and be in health, even as thy soul prospereth." I realized I had studied training, but failed to study enough on the nutritional part. Now I realize if I had my P.E.R Fat Loss System, I would not have gained that weight back. So when people say you have to eat right, do they know what that mean? When we tell people to eat right we leave it up to them to define what is eating right. I found that there is a science to eating based on the individual body type and what they want to accomplish. Do they want an athletic build, body builder's build, or do they just want to obtain health? Some people may look healthy because of their body types, which can be very deceiving. There are three body types: endomorph, mesomorph, and ectomorph. The endomorph gains weight very easy, while the mesomorph has a great physique and appears to work out. However, working out is not necessary to maintain their physique simply because of their genetic makeup. Last we have the ectomorph which are those who seem to eat everything and not gain weight at all. I have all body types on my P.E.R. Fat Loss System because the person may not appear to be fat on the outside, but they are "fat" on the inside. Believe it or not, there are some 150 pound adults whose insides are more damaged than those who weigh 450 pounds. Although obesity is an epidemic and dangerous to your health, those smaller in frame think they are healthier because of their size and that's not entirely true. There are people who suffer from hypertension, diabetes, high cholesterol, etc. in each body type group.

4

WORDS OF MOTIVATION

2 Tim 2:15 "Study to show thyself approved unto God, a workman that needs not to be ashamed, rightly dividing the word of truth."

- Study to show, not just to know.
- When you know why you are doing, what you are doing then you can repeat it at will.

NOTES

_____

_____

_____

_____

_____

_____

_____

_____

_____

CHAPTER 2
THE DETERMINING FACTOR

We must be responsible in the areas in which we want to succeed, you must have knowledge. 1 Thess 4:4 "That every one of you should know how to possess his vessel in sanctification and honor." According to the scripture, to possess your vessel you have to know something and to know something means you have to learn something. The subject I focused on was my health and I wanted to know how to make my body work with me rather than against me. There are three different body types and it is essential to know your body type and what works for you. The determining factor to my success was studying my body type and how my body functions. I have heard people say they are determined to lose weight and they are quite diligent in the beginning; only to experience temporary or no results. When desired results are not seen quickly, most will quit. However, determination without knowledge will soon diminish.

Hormonal imbalances also play a role and work against your body. Examples include: ghrelin which is the appetite inducing hormone; leptin which decreases your appetite and communicates to your brain when you are full; insulin which is secreted from the pancreas and can cause your body to store fat; and glucagon which is secreted from the pancreas also when there is a sufficient amount of protein and will cause the body to use stored body fat for energy. When these hormones are unstable and they don't function properly, you may find yourself hungry 15 minutes after eating dinner. These hormonal imbalances can cause your body to work against your health and weight lose goals. What causes these hormones to be out of whack? The answer is simple; the foods we eat are injected with hormones and the vegetables are sprayed with pesticides. These are just a few things that can cause hormonal imbalance and until these issues are addressed you will continue to fight a losing battle when it comes to losing weight. That's why my P.E.R. Fat Loss System is imperative in addressing these issues so your body can submit and you can finally succeed in getting your weight and health goals accomplished.

Every year individuals across the world make that New Year's weight loss resolution, only to fall off after a few weeks. If you get the solution, you will not need another resolution or redo what you failed at before. Proverbs 4:7 "Wisdom is the principal thing; therefore get wisdom: and with all thy getting get understanding."

When you obtain and execute wisdom knowledge and understanding, then you are on your way to success. When you have a system that is giving you the results you desire and you understand how you did it, you can repeat it at will and that encourages you to remain on course. Obtaining the wisdom is essential because you will then know why you are doing what you are doing. Then and only then can you maintain continued success.

Confronting Hormonal Issues: When your hormones are out of whack you will experience a loss of energy and mental clarity. Digestion problems affect your metabolism, libido, you will experience a loss of lean muscle mass, increased belly fat, and problems with your skin complexion. That's why my P.E.R. Fat Loss System is designed to balance hormones because I combine the right protein, carbohydrates, and healthy fats. All of these are critical in balancing hormones. When there is hormonal balance it will destroy food cravings, increase energy, give you glowing skin, increased fertility, stable your mood, and you will also experience the body's ability to heal itself.

WORDS OF MOTIVATION

Prov 10:4 "He becometh poor that dealeth with a slack hand: but the hand of the diligent maketh rich."

Procrastination is the assassination of the motivation necessary for momentum, mobilization and manifestation.

NOTES

_____

_____

_____

_____

_____

_____

_____

_____

_____

_____

_____

CHAPTER 3
THE GREAT COMEBACK

There is nothing better than seeing your favorite team playing and at one point they are losing, but all of a sudden something kicks in. Their drive becomes noticeable, their attitude changes, and something kicks in giving them a desire to win. Something kicks in causing a reverse in the games flow and your team begins to comeback. Then you witness it, crunch time, and they shout out "Leave it all on the field!" In the last minute they come out victorious. That is what I need you to do; get rid of all the negativity, doubt and past failures. You asked for it, you prayed for it, and you have made certain confessions for your health and longevity. Now the answer is here and all I want you to do is leave it all on the field.

In this chapter of my life I am 48 years old, my health is diminishing, I am on blood pressure medicine, my cholesterol is high, and for six months I have been getting up six to seven times a night going to the restroom. I hoped these symptoms would pass; however, after a period of time with no change, I decided it needed a doctor's attention. When I went to the doctor he ran various tests. The test results were quite surprising, everything was normal. I was not relieved, but instead somewhat confused. I do not have the education these doctors have and I certainly do not have a PhD, but I did know something was totally wrong with my body. I prayed to God for insight and the Spirit of God spoke to my heart saying, "Are you going to listen to the doctors or your body?" My response was, "They know more than I know." God said, "I know more than them, the student is never greater than the teacher." God instructed me to combine particular foods to eat, and after eating this combination of foods I went to sleep. That night, much to my amazement, I did not get up one time. I was so excited I decided to try this food combination another five days and as a result my cholesterol went back to normal, I was taken off of blood pressure medicine, and my eye sight went back to 20/20. That is when I realized God has given us food to heal the body. I continued with this way of eating and unbeknownst to me I was losing a massive amount of weight. Over the course of the next two or three weeks my suits began to look baggy/saggy. I was losing weight at a rate of 35lbs in 21 days to 54lbs in 42 days. I went from a 48 waist to a 32 waist in that same amount of time. The quality of my life changed, my energy level went through the roof, and my sleep at night was incredible. I was ecstatic because God had given me the secret to living a healthy lifestyle.

Words of Motivation

2 Cor 2:14 "Now thanks be unto God, which always causeth us to triumph in Christ, and maketh manifest the savour of his knowledge by us in every place."

"We win from within", "There is no failure in Christ"

NOTES

_____

_____

_____

_____

_____

_____

_____

_____

_____

_____

_____

_____

_____

_____

_____

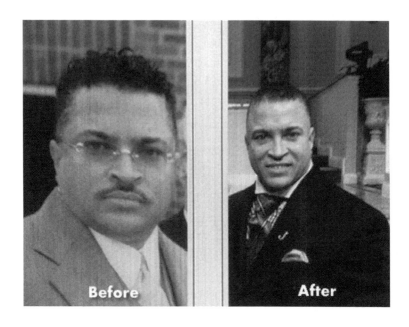

CHAPTER 4
FAT LOSS VS. WEIGHT LOSS

Are you losing the right kind of weight?

This is a crucial question simply because there are people who are losing weight, but they are losing the wrong weight. They are losing muscle mass rather than body fat and you can usually recognize these individuals because they look frail, have loose skin, and sometimes even have a skeletal appearance. On my P.E.R. Fat Loss System it targets body fat so as you lose weight (body fat not muscle mass), you will possess that vibrant healthy appearance throughout the process.

I try to encourage people on my plan to stay off the scale after the first initial weigh-in. This is because in my fat loss system we target fat while maintaining and developing muscle mass. If you lose 3 pounds of fat and have gained 3 pounds of muscle, your weight will not change, but you have lost an inch in your waist. Here is another example: you have two men both are

6'2 at 220. One looks like a machine and the other looks like a barrow; what's the difference between the two? One's body fat percentage is higher than the other. I tell clients just because you lose weight does not mean you are losing the right kind of weight.

You must first understand there is a difference between fat loss and weight loss. My P.E.R. Fat Loss System is the proper eating regimen (a specific combinations of protein, low glycemic carbohydrates and healthy fats) that targets fat rather than muscle and helps maintain and develop muscle. Weight loss is when people lose body fat and muscle mass. That creates a big problem and can cause health challenges. My fat loss system targets body fat while maintaining muscle mass, so as you are losing fat you can preserve a healthy vibrant look and continue a healthy lifestyle.

The day you start the P.E.R. Fat Loss System is the day your body stops storing fat, and you will learn how to burn the stored body fat you presently have. This will primarily be accomplished through nutrition, knowing what to eat on a day-to-day bases, and also what to eat before and after your workout. Remember learn to trust the process not the scale because when you continue you will get the desired outcome you so desire and they will be permanent.

WORDS OF MOTIVATION

Proverbs 13:20 "He that walketh with wise men shall be wise: but a companion of fools shall be destroyed."

- Your imagination needs the stimulation and association of successful others.

Notes

_____

_____

_____

_____

_____

_____

_____

_____

_____

_____

_____

_____

_____

_____

_____

_____

_____

_____

_____

_____

_____

_____

_____

_____

_____

CHAPTER 5

CREATING A STRONG WHY

To know if a person will succeed in any area, rather it be goals, vision, or dreams, ask them this question, "Why are you doing this?" I often find that if a person's "why" is not strong enough their drive won't last.

Your "why" must be strong in your succeeding on this P.E.R. Fat Loss System. If your only desire is to get in a size thirty four jeans or a size six dress, that might get you there. Unfortunately, that has been proven not to be enough motivation to keep you there. However, if you enter into this endeavor with a desire to be healthy or increase the quality of your life, then you are more likely to be committed to stay on course and continue with the plan making it a successful lifestyle. The next key is when you start on this plan you need to go in with the right attitude. Do not say "I am going to try it out" you need to say "I am going to do it" and trust the process. I had individuals that said, "I know someone that tried your plan and it did not work for them." With a 90% success rate I told her, "Wow! That's funny that with all those succeeding on my system you would have to find the failure. And what concerns me is how easy it is for you to relate to the 10% failure rate rather than the 90% of those that succeeded. This system has been tried and proven. I do not make guarantees, but I have enough clients to prove my system works. There are doctors, dietitians, and fitness trainers that are on my plan. When you want to live and experience a better quality of life, this plan is for you."

We are responsible for our health and we can make these confessions of the 120 club coming from the scripture Gen 6:3, "And the Lord said, my spirit shall not always strive with man, for that he also is flesh: yet his days shall be an hundred and twenty years." Even though it's a promise, most people are not living to this age, instead they are dying prematurely. There is no one sounding the alarm so I am stepping up to sound it. There are items we purchase that have been approved to sit on the grocer's shelves, directly working against our longevity and quality of life. We need to be more responsible and educate ourselves on what we are putting into our bodies. There are foods on our grocer's shelves that are proven to be addictive, some that cause hormonal imbalance, and some that contribute to heart disease and diabetes. When we struggle with our weight we have to remember, it is not entirely our fault. We are eating foods that's been approved by the food industry that causes us to crave more foods. The secret to succeeding on the outside is we must confront the challenges on the inside:

- Hormonal imbalances
- Food cravings
- Health challenges
- Lack of energy
- Sleep deprivation

Here are some other health challenges our clients were healed from:

- Hypertension
- High Cholesterol
- Diabetes
- Erectile Dysfunction

WORDS OF MOTIVATION

Proverbs 13:4 "The soul of the sluggard desireth, and hath nothing: but the soul of the diligent shall be made fat."

- The diligent shall be rewarded
- Lazy people want what you have, but don't want to do what you do.

NOTES

_____

_____

_____

_____

_____

_____

_____

_____

_____

_____

_____

_____

_____

_____

_____

_____

_____

_____

CHAPTER 6

THE SCIENCE OF EATING

We have heard the phrase, "Out of sight, out of mind" and I realize when people cannot see the damage that certain foods do in their body it really does not concern them until it's too late, they get sick, or get that bad report from the doctor. My job is to open the eyes of my clients so they can know the effects certain foods have on the body by allowing them to see it on the canvas of their imagination so they can visualize what is occurring in their body. When you start my P.E.R. Fat Loss System eating will become an experience. You will understand what you ate to experience a burst of energy and also you will know what you ate that causes you to feel sluggish.

To get from fat to fit I used my P.E.R. Fat Loss System, which is knowing the right food combination designed to heal the body and target body fat rather than muscle mass. We will start with the five day body slam which is a combination of proteins and low glycemic complex carbohydrates while drinking lemon water and vinegar. The lemon water and vinegar mixture will immediately stop your blood sugar from spiking, keeping your body from going into fat storing mode, along with a host of other benefits.

After the five day body slam we move directly to the P.E.R. Plan menu which consists of proteins, low glycemic complex carbohydrates, and healthy fats. All play an essential part in continuing the fat loss process while maintaining and developing muscle mass. It is one process to stop your body from storing fat, but it is another process to teach your body to burn the stored body fat that it currently has. Your body does not automatically use stored body fat for energy because it is really designed to hold on to body fat in case of sickness that may result in fat loss. Most of us have way too much reserved body fat and we have to eat the right combinations of food to activate the hormone glucagon. This hormone communicates to your body to use stored body fat for energy rather than stripping from your muscles and organs trying to obtain energy. When you work out, follow the food combining fat loss system, and target only the body fat instead of the muscle mass, then you will see and get permanent results.

Taking a closer look at the hormone glucagon: Glucagon works differently than insulin and it is known as the fat burning hormone. The pancreas hormone, insulin, is released once your blood sugar has spiked because of moderate or high glycemic carbohydrates and it pulls fat from the blood stream and stores it as fat, but the hormone glucagon is stimulated because of a sufficient amount of protein. Glucagon main purpose is to maintain blood sugar and use stored body fat as energy.

There are those that found, as a result of them getting their nutrition in order, they no longer suffered from a sleep disorder. When we go to sleep at night just because we are sleep doesn't mean our bodies have stopped working. Our body needs energy and because you have not eaten the right combination before you went to bed your body is now struggling while you are trying to sleep to find energy and this can disrupt your sleep. When numerous clients started the P.E.R. Fat Loss System one of the first things they noticed was how sound their sleep was and how refreshed they were in the morning. This is simply because when you eat the right combination before you go to bed, your body can use stored body fat for energy and stop interfering with your sleep time.

WORDS OF MOTIVATION

Heb 6:12 "That ye be not slothful, but followers of them who through faith and patience inherit the promises."

- Patience, Process and Promise
- The power to imitate is the power to duplicate

NOTES

_____

_____

_____

_____

_____

_____

_____

_____

_____

_____

_____

_____

_____

_____

_____

_____

_____

_____

_____

_____

CHAPTER 7

UNDERSTANDING THE GLYCEMIC INDEX

Understanding is a major key in succeeding in any area and when you understand why you are doing what you are doing then you can repeat it at will. So me studying this for myself was the difference between success and failure. It's alright to take advice from individuals, but a least go and research what they told you to see if it is true.

On my P.E.R. Fat Loss System we eat low glycemic complex carbohydrates the majority of the time, which are fruits and vegetables for fiber, and we stay away from starchy complex carbohydrates. It is important that you research what low glycemic complex carbohydrates you need. Now let me give you a better understanding of the glycemic index it is the effect the carbohydrates have on blood sugar levels after consumption. When you eat high glycemic carbohydrates, it causes your blood sugar to spike, the pancreas to release the hormone insulin that pulls the fat from the blood stream, and it causes your body to go into fat storing mode. That is why it is important to know which carbohydrates will maintain stable blood sugar levels. The levels to be mindful of on the glycemic index are low, medium and high carbohydrates numbers. So 55 and less is considered low, medium is 56 to 69, and high glycemic carbohydrates are 70 and above. You want to eat low glycemic complex carbohydrates. as much as possible. If you happen to eat medium or high glycemic complex carbohydrates be sure to eat them in combination with a low glycemic carbohydrate to counter the effect of the medium or high glycemic carbohydrate to stop or minimize any fat storing.

What I've learned about juicing: *I don't encourage juicing simply because you will not do it the rest of your life and most people do not educate themselves before they begin juicing. Losing weight is not a problem,* *anybody can lose weight juicing, but can you keep it off and are you losing the right weight? Are you losing muscle or body fat? Well let me answer that for you, you are losing muscle and it will not be long before it comes back as fat. The problem with this is you need protein to maintain muscle mass and because you extract the pulp from the fruit and vegetables it causes your blood sugar to spike and your body goes into fat storing mode. The pulp in the juice is what helps to keep your blood sugar stabilized and stop the fat storing process. So think before you drink.*

The truth about detoxing: *I believe in detoxing the body as a matter of fact the first five days of my system, The Body Slam, is a detox and it is designed to rid the body of toxin and is capable of getting a body that is out of order back in order. However, there are dangers with long term detoxing that can result in mineral and vitamin deficiencies. That is why any doctor will tell you do not detox no longer than 3-5 days.*

How to Prevent Plateau: *Plateau is when your body has become accustomed to the workout and you have minimal or no weight loss results and that's why you should always do various workouts. Another way to break a plateau is by my Yo-Yo cycling, which is food manipulation. That's when I instruct the clients after eating from the P.E.R.'s menu for 30-60 days they must increase their caloric intake by eating a high calorie meal, including dessert. When you eat a high calorie meal it increases your metabolism and jumpstarts your body to start losing body fat. Some may consider this a cheat day, but I don't call it a cheat day simply because a cheat day is designed to take care of a craving, but on my system, the P.E.R. Fat Loss System, it strips you of your food cravings.*

On my P.E.R. Fat Loss System I encourage everyone to work out as your energy increases, but working out without a proper nutritional guideline will produce minimal to no results. Nutrition is 70% to you succeeding your ultimate fat and weight loss goals and working out is 30%, but it will accelerate the fat loss process. So keep this in mind while on your journey. I have workout tips toward the end of the book. Let's get started today!

WORDS OF MOTIVATION

Prov 11:14 "Where no counsel is, the people fall: but in the multitude of counselors there is safety."

- Association produces assimilation
- Actions reveal your knowledge or lack of knowledge
- Associate with those that know more than you, otherwise you will not be any better than you are right now.

NOTES

_____

_____

_____

_____

_____

_____

_____

_____

_____

_____

_____

_____

_____

_____

_____

_____

_____

_____

_____

_____

_____

_____

_____

_____

_____

Sample menu:

Breakfast:
Eggs
Turkey Bacon/Sausage
Oatmeal
Fruit

Snack:
Trail mix

Lunch:
Grilled Chicken/ Fish
Asparagus

Snacks:
Protein drink
Fruit

Dinner:
Rotisserie Chicken
Salad (Vinaigrette dressing)

Dessert:
Greek Yogurt

Workout Regimen

Sunday: Rest

Monday: Full Body Resistant Band
Workout

Tuesday: Walking (1 hour)

Wednesday: Full Body Weight
LiftingWorkout

Thursday: Walking (1 hour)

Friday: Full Body Workout

Saturday: Walking (1 hour)

Bonus/Alternate Workout Tips:

Biking: Stationary
Biking: Actual Aerobics
Running: Treadmill
Running: Road
Running: Just Hills
Walking: Brisk
Stair Climber
Swimming

FYI: *All workouts should be at least an hour long*

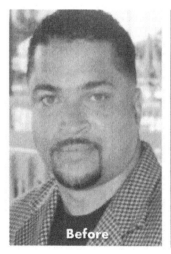 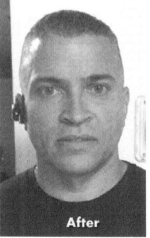

BONUS:
WORDS OF MOTIVATION

Prov 23:7 "For as he thinketh in his heart, so is he: Eat and drink, saith he to thee; but his heart is not with thee."

- The quality of your life is determined by the quality of your thinking.
- Whatever you believe will become your reality.

Gal 6:9 "And let us not be weary in well doing: for in due season we shall reap, if we faint not."

- Possessing the tenacity to hold your course.
- Hope in future results produce perseverance in the present.

2 Tim 4:7 "I have fought a good fight, I have finished my course, I have kept the faith"

- Starting is good; finishing is better
- Don't lose your fight
- The power of determination

Jer 29:11 "For I know the thoughts that I think toward you, saith the Lord, thoughts of peace, and not of evil, to give you an expected end."

- The power of the end result
- Determination always has a vision in sight

Isa 46:10 "Declaring the end from the beginning."

- See yourself there before you get the
- See yourself as a winner before you start

Rom 4:17 "And calleth those things which be not as though they were."

- Framing your future with the words of your mouth
- If you are not saying anything you are not creating anything

Prov 18:21 "Death and life are in the power of the tongue: and they that love it shall eat the fruit thereof."

- Speaking life over your visions, goals and dreams
- Don't sabotage your goals by the words of your mouth

Deut 30:19 "I call heaven and earth to record this day against you, that I have set before you life and death, blessing and cursing: therefore choose life, that both thou and thy seed may live."

- Choose life that destroys generational curses
- Leave a legacy of life for the generations to come

Hebrews 11:1 "Now faith is the substance of things hoped for, the evidence of things not seen."

- Faith is living in a future hope that's so real it gives absolute assurance in the present
- You got to see it before you see it
- You got to be it before you be it

Acts 17:11 "These were nobler than those in Thessalonica, in that they received the word with all readiness of mind, and searched the scriptures daily, whether those things were so."

- When you study for yourself then there is no one else to blame
- If you succeed it's your fault, if you fail it's your fault

Proverbs 21:5 "Good planning and hard work lead to prosperity, but hasty shortcuts lead to poverty."

- Set yourself to win
- Success is not by accident.
- You succeed on purpose

Gen 6:3 "And the Lord said, My spirit shall not always strive with man, for that he also is flesh: yet his days shall be a hundred and twenty years."

- Do not cheat yourself out of life.
- When you die prematurely you rob society of your impacting inspiring purpose.

Testimonial

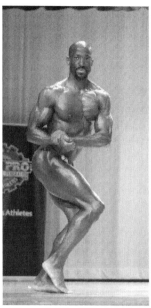

My Name is Darryl K. Washington Sr. I am a Lifetime Natural Bodybuilder. When I heard about the PER Plan I was very curious and wondered what it was all about! As a Natural Bodybuilder losing weight was not my challenge but Bodybuilding is about the "Extreme"! Getting Extremely Lean can take a toll on your hormones! I had the opportunity to use Chandler Coleman's PER and I was very impressed with both the way it made me feel (I had super energy) and that it enabled my body (hormones) to reset itself! I would highly recommend the PER Plan to anyone looking to regain and take control of their health! The first week alone is worth the price of the PER Plan!

Testimonial
Tasha Estep

Starting Weight: 205 lbs

After losing 50 lbs - Ending Weight: 155lbs

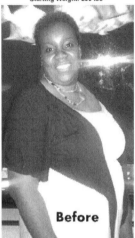

Before

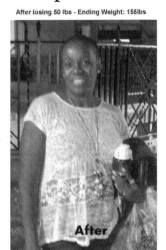

After

I began my journey with Chandler Coleman's PER Plan in September of 2011. I started the plan ready for a change. During that time, it became very important to me to lose weight and obtain optimum health for the benefit of my infant daughter and my family. Prior to meeting with Mr. Coleman to obtain information about his PER Plan, I was experiencing a slight numbing in my right arm and leg when laying down which prompted me to start doing Zumba 3 days a week. I was beginning to feel great, but did not obtain any real reduction in my weight due to inadequate food choices. The first 3 days were the toughest for me because it challenged my thoughts about food and also challenged me to eat differently. I realized after day 1 that my current approach to food was defeating my daily attempts at working out and losing weight. The wonderful thing about this PER plan is that it also revealed that I was allergic to dairy and was sensitive to foods that contained gluten. Thus, attention to food labels and food choices were critical for me.

On our meeting day, I was wearing a size 14/16 in plus sizes. Within the first 30 days, I went from a size 14/16 down to a size 10. At that time not only did the numbing stop, I found myself with more energy for my family, I awoke well rested due to better sound sleep at night, and I began varying and increasing my daily workouts in the gym. During this process, I did not weigh myself on the scale regularly but I did submit facial photos every few weeks to Mr. Coleman to reveal my new leaner size. Within 6 months I was down to a size 6, had a smaller abdominal area and was very much involved in my new healthy fit lifestyle. To date, almost 3 years later, I continue to maintain my size 6 using the same information obtained on day one from Mr. Coleman. In addition to pursuing the very best that the PER Plan had to offer, I have also coupled my new found zeal for my healthy lifestyle with successfully obtaining my certification as a Spinning Instructor in which I teach daily in a local gym.

Thanks Mr. Coleman for hearing the voice of God and obeying. My life and the life of others around me is that much greater!

Testimonial

My name is Anthony Minor I am 54 years old and have been on Chandler Coleman's P.E.R. Fat Loss System for the last two years. I thank God for Mr. Coleman not only did the program help me lose weight but it has given me a new lease on life and living a better quality of life. The program has afforded me the opportunity to get off my hypertension medication and brought my diabetes concern to naught. My energy levels are extremely high and having the knowledge I received from Mr. Coleman's system has empowered me to maintain my desire fat loss and weight goals for over 2 years. When I started the P.E.R. Fat Loss System I weighed in at 262 pounds and after 90 days I am at 198 pounds, I was a 47 in the waist and that went to a 35 in the same amount of time.

Testimonial

I visited Chandler last summer June 2013 and he introduced me to an unique program called Lifestyle INC P.E.R Fat loss System. I been in the health and wellness business for over 20 years as a personal trainer and fitness director and studied a number of food plans and diets, but never experienced a plan as simple and effective as Chandlers P.E.R plan. I started his program weighting 236lbs and lost 10bs of BODYFAT in the 1st week 226lbs and another 16lbs in the following 2 weeks. But what was most impressive was the over physical and energy enhancement that was phenomenal, I also went from a 40 inch waist to 35 inches. His science is second to none in my opinion. I am currently living in Arizona and have a sports performance company and health and wellness gym and have all my clients using his techniques.

Larry Graham CPT.

FAT 2 FIT Quick Tips

Eating Tips:

1. Drink plenty of water. Your body needs a lot of water so give in to water. Water is not just a way to flush out toxin but if you have more water in your body you will generally feel healthier and fuller. This itself will discourage any tendency to gorge.

2. Stay away from sweetened bottle drinks, especially sodas. Hey all those colas and fizzy drinks are sweetened with sugar and sugar means calories. The more you can cut out on these sweetened bottle drinks, the better for you. So if you must drink sodas, then stick to diet sodas.

3. Eat low glycemic fruit instead of drinking fruit juice. Juice is often sweetened but fresh fruits have natural sugars. When you eat low glycemic fruit, you are taking in a lot of

fiber, which is needed by the body, and fruits of course are an excellent source of vitamins.

4. Start your day with a glass of water. As soon as you wake up, gulp down a glass of cool water. It's a wonderful way to start you day and you only need a lesser quantity of your breakfast drink after that. Drink a gallon of water a day.

5. Choose low glycemic fruit to processed fruits. Processed and canned fruits do not have as much fiber as fresh fruit and processed and canned fruits are nearly always sweetened.

6. Increase your fiber intake. Like I mentioned, the body needs a lot of fiber. So try to include in your diet as many low glycemic fruits and vegetables as you can.

7. Stay on the P.E.R. eating regimen don't deviate unless it's during yo-yo cycling. Keep a watchful eye on everything that goes in. Sometimes the garnishes and sauces can be

richer than the food itself.

8. Only snack on those given on the P.E.R. plan menu and they are counted as meals also so that can help to keep the body fueled,

9. I allow people to drink tea and coffee black, unless sweeten with the recommended sweeteners (no creamers), however be mindful that caffeine can constrict blood vessels that can hinder the blood flow. I have a food combination that dilate blood vessel and purifies the blood for maximum blood flow that will help in the area of increased energy.

10. Stay away from fried things. The unhealthy high saturated fat contain in fried chicken, fried fish, even fried eggs will directly interfere with your quality of life and longevity When you avoid fried foods then you avoid free radical which are unpaired electrons that attach themselves to healthy cells and destroys them.

11. Make dark chocolate (1once per serving) a luxury and not a routine. It is good for heart health just do not indulge too much in it.

12. It's always best to have a P.E.R. Plan breakfast before walking so that your body can charge itself with the energy it needs. Breakfast is the most important meal of the day, but that does not mean that it should be the most filling meal of the day.

13. Low glycemic vegetables are better raw or steamed lightly than cooked or canned vegetables. When you cook them, you are in fact taking away nearly half the vitamins and nutrients in them. When you buy your vegetables try organic that is pesticide free.

14. Train yourself to always have your food prepared ahead of time. Try to have food at fixed times of the day.

15. Vinegar and lemon water have incredible benefits to help your body to comply to what you want to accomplish.

16. Develop a habit of chewing all food at least 8 to 12 times. This is essential to add saliva to the food and help in the digestion process.

17. Choose low fat substitutes or no fat substitutes. There are plenty of low fat or even no fat substitutes available in the market so why not choose wisely.

18. Use a nonstick frying pan for your cooking and if you have to use oil use Smart Balance butter or Pam.

19. Always combine protein and low glycemic carbohydrates (fiber based and avoid starchy) so after your body depletes the energy from the carbohydrates, it's the protein that activates the fat burning hormone glucagon.

20. Remember I eat until I go to bed but avoid high glycemic carbohydrates because that will turn to stored body fat simply

because of that need to be burned off. Rather eat protein and or low glycemic carbohydrates so your body can burn fat while you sleep.

SOME OF THE MOST COMMONLY ASKED QUESTIONS

Q. Is it safe to lose 54 pounds in 42 days?
A. Number one, it depends on what kind of weight you are losing, muscle or body fat, and number 2, if you are sick or not. If you are not sick and you are losing body fat and not muscle then absolutely it is very safe.

Q. How do you know if you are losing muscle or body fat?
A. I use a fat loss monitor because a scale can tell you your weight, but it can't tell you your lean-fat ratio. To be sure you are losing fat and not muscle a scale cannot help, you need a fat loss monitor.

Q. If you lose that much weight that fast won't it come back fast?
A. Once again if you are losing muscle rather than body fat yes, but 90% of my folks have not gained any back because we are losing body fat and maintaining and developing muscle and for some it's been over 2 years

and nothing has come back.

Q. Do I have to take a special drink or pills?
A. No, if you are talking about weight loss supplements, absolutely not. My system is all natural food combining to accomplish my goals. I do encourage clients to take vitamins.

Q. Who would best benefit from the P.E.R. Fat Loss System?
A. Those who want to be healthy or maintain their health. I have clients from 100 pounds to 500 pounds and just because an individual's weight is ideal does not mean they are healthy or other areas do not need to be addressed.

Q. Women ask "Will I be built like a man?"
A. Because I talk about body fat loss while maintaining muscle mass women think that will cause them to look muscular, and that is absolutely not true. While it is important to maintain muscle mass because as you lose body fat you do not want saggy hanging skin,

nor scrawny necks. This system is designed so that no matter how much weight you lose you can maintain a toned healthy vibrant appearance.

Q. Can children do it?
A. Usually after an evaluation I can determine that, but if they can't do the Body Slam they definitely can do the P.E.R. Plan menu and get great results.

Q. Can elderly folks do it?
A. Absolutely, I have quite a few older individuals and they say it feels like they have a new lease on life, but I instruct everyone to inform their doctors of any weight loss system they start.

Q. Can I eat my favorite foods?
A. I do. That's where my food combining comes in, so I can show you what foods to combine with your favorite foods so that those foods that will usually cause your body

to go into fat storing mode won't.

Q. How much does it cost?
A. HOW MUCH ARE YOU WORTH?

WE WOULD LOVE TO HEAR FROM YOU!

VISIT OUR WEBSITE
chandlercoleman.com

EMAIL US @
pcoleman7@verizon.net

Facebook
Chandler Coleman

Instagram
mybarberpc

Follow me on Twitter
Chandler

32768744R00042

Made in the USA
Lexington, KY
01 June 2014